PSORIASIS

Discovery of Psoriasis: Causes, Diagnosis, and Methods for Patient-Centered Dermatological Treatment

CHAD BRUNO

Table of Contents

Introductory

Rapid accumulation of skin cells on the skin's surface is a symptom of psoriasis, a persistent skin disorder. Thick, silvery scales and itchy, dry, red spots that can be unpleasant result from this accumulation of dead skin cells. Psoriasis is an autoimmune disorder in which the body's immune system inappropriately attacks healthy skin cells, leading to their rapid proliferation.

• Although the specific cause of psoriasis is unknown, it is thought that both hereditary and environmental factors play a role.

Some people may only have modest symptoms, while others may suffer from debilitating conditions that severely disrupt their daily lives.

• Elbows, knees, scalp, face, palms, and soles are just few of the places psoriasis can appear. In addition to the physical symptoms, psoriasis can also have psychological and emotional impacts on those who suffer from it, as it can be cosmetically upsetting and may lead to social and self-esteem concerns.

Combinations of oral medications, topical creams, phototherapy (light therapy), and sometimes biologic drugs that target specific immune system components are used to treat psoriasis. Treatment tries to lessen the symptoms, slow the rapid skin cell proliferation, and control the illness efficiently. The intensity and type of a person's psoriasis may dictate how they are treated. Psoriasis sufferers need to collaborate with medical experts to create an individualized treatment strategy.

CHAPTER ONE
Analyzing the Past

Psoriasis has been known about for millennia and its symptoms have been reported in various ways throughout that time. Consider the following background information on psoriasis:

• Psoriasis has a long history, going back thousands of years and mentioned in ancient scriptures and medical works. Psoriasis is thought to have existed even in ancient times; it was mentioned by the ancient Egyptians. In fact, the word "psoriasis" comes from the

Greek word "psora," which means "itch."

- Psoriasis was linked to many different myths and beliefs throughout medieval Europe. It was considered a curse or a punishment by some. At times, those who suffered with psoriasis faced social isolation and prejudice.

- As medical science advanced throughout the 19th century, so did our knowledge of psoriasis. In the middle of the nineteenth century, Austrian dermatologist Ferdinand von Hebra invented the term "psoriasis" to describe a skin condition. He noticed the particular characteristics of the illness and distinguished it from other skin disorders.

• Research into psoriasis had a dramatic uptick in the 20th century. The role of the immune system in this disease was better understood by medical practitioners. New alternatives for the treatment and control of psoriasis emerged with the development of topical and systemic therapies including corticosteroids and phototherapy.

• **Current Times:** Psoriasis research and knowledge have made great strides in the last few decades. Researchers have made great strides in understanding the immunological and genetic mechanisms that contribute to psoriasis. Because of this, more specific and efficient therapies, such as biologic medicines, have emerged.

In addition, initiatives to educate the public about psoriasis and lessen the stigma that surrounds it have gained traction. Psoriasis research and education have benefited by the establishment of advocacy groups and organizations that provide emotional and practical assistance to people with psoriasis.

Psoriasis is still incurable, but there are better treatment choices than ever before. Research efforts are ongoing to better understand the causes of psoriasis and develop more effective treatments for the condition. Looking back at psoriasis through the ages sheds light on how far our knowledge and ability to treat this complicated skin condition have come.

Types of Psoriasis

Psoriasis is a complicated disease with a number of subtypes, each with its unique set of signs and symptoms. Psoriasis can manifest itself in five main forms:

1. Eighty percent to ninety percent of all psoriasis cases are classified as plaque psoriasis.

Plaques are elevated, red areas of skin that are coated in thick, silvery-white scales.

The elbows, knees, lower back, and scalp are common areas for these plaques to manifest.

2. Psoriasis guttate:

• A bacterial or viral illness, like streptococcal throat infection, is usually what sets off guttate psoriasis.

Tiny, teardrop-shaped, red or pink patches appear on the skin.

• Guttate psoriasis is a common skin condition among young people.

3. Psoriasis with a twist:

• Skin folds (armpits, groin, beneath the breasts, and between the buttocks) are common places for inverse psoriasis to manifest as red, smooth, and shiny lesions.

• The increased pain and discomfort is likely attributable to the increased skin-on-skin friction in these locations.

4. Inflammatory Skin Disease with Pustules

• Pustules, or small blisters, filled with pus, characterize pustular psoriasis.

Palmoplantar pustulosis (which affects the palms and soles) and generalized pustular psoriasis (which affects the entire body) are two types of pustular psoriasis.

The severity of this rare kind of psoriasis is high.

5. Red Psoriasis of the Skin:

• Rare yet severe, erythrodermic psoriasis causes extreme redness and skin loss over extensive portions of the body.

Extreme itching, agony, and the potential for problems including dehydration and infection are all possible side effects.

• Medical attention must be sought right away for erythrodermic psoriasis.

Psoriasis comes in a variety of subtypes, some of which are more uncommon and poorly understood than others. These include nail psoriasis (which affects fingernails and toenails), scalp psoriasis (which occurs on the scalp), and psoriatic arthritis (an inflammatory form of arthritis that is sometimes associated with psoriasis).

Individuals with the same psoriasis diagnosis may experience a wide range in symptom severity. It is crucial to see a dermatologist or other medical professional if you experience symptoms of psoriasis or suspect you have the condition.

CHAPTER TWO
Reasons & Prompts

Although the root causes of psoriasis are yet unknown, environmental and genetic factors are thought to play a role. The following are some of the hypothesized causes and aggravating factors of psoriasis:

1. Psoriasis tends to run in families; hence heredity is a major factor in its onset. Children of psoriatic parents are more likely to develop the skin problem themselves. Psoriasis has been linked to specific genes.

2. Because the immune system incorrectly identifies and assaults healthy skin cells, psoriasis is classified as an autoimmune disease. White blood cells known as T cells are suspected to play a pivotal role in this immunological reaction.

3. Psoriasis in individuals who have a genetic predisposition can be triggered or made worse by a number of environmental variables.

Guttate psoriasis can be triggered or made worse by bacterial or viral illnesses such streptococcal throat infections.

- Injury or Trauma: In some situations, physical trauma to the skin, such as cuts, burns, or sunburn, can induce the development of psoriasis in that location. The name for this is the Koebner phenomenon.

- **Stress:** For some people, emotional stress is a precipitating factor in the development of psoriasis or a worsening of their existing symptoms.

Some medications, including lithium, antimalarial treatments, and beta-blockers, have been linked to either causing psoriasis or making the condition worse.

There is a correlation between psoriasis and the use of tobacco products and heavy alcohol intake.

4. Some people's psoriasis flare-ups are made worse by fluctuations in their hormone levels, which can happen during times like pregnancy and menopause.

5. Excess body fat is linked to inflammation, which may exacerbate psoriasis symptoms, and obesity is thought to exacerbate the illness.

6. Some people with psoriasis report that their symptoms improve when the weather is warm and sunny, and worsen when the weather is cold and dry.

7. Although dietary adjustments may be helpful in controlling psoriasis, the available scientific evidence is inconclusive. But for some, eating particular foods or being exposed to foods that cause an allergic reaction might actually bring on or exacerbate symptoms.

It's crucial to keep in mind that the causes of psoriasis might differ from person to person. What exacerbates the illness in one individual may not impact another. Psoriasis can be managed and controlled with a mix of medical treatments and alterations to one's lifestyle, including the identification and avoidance of personal triggers. It is essential to see a doctor for a diagnosis and individualized treatment plan if you suspect you have psoriasis or are experiencing symptoms.

Problems with Psoriasis

Psoriasis is a long-term skin disorder with a wide range of possible manifestations. Depending on the kind and severity of the psoriasis, the individual has a wide range of symptoms.

1. Plaques are scaly, elevated regions of skin that can be either red or pink in color. The most common kind of psoriasis is characterized by these plaques.

2. Itching is a common symptom of psoriasis and can be very bothersome.

3. Color Change to Red or Pink: The damaged skin is often a deeper shade of red or pink than the surrounding healthy skin.

4. Excessive cell turnover of the skin causes a silvery white scaling to form on and around the plaques. These scales have been known to shed and cling to whatever they land on.

5. Plaques from psoriasis often look dry, and they can crack or bleed if they are rubbed or scratched.

6. Inflammation: Psoriasis is connected with skin inflammation. It's possible to get a warm skin sensation in some circumstances.

7. Psoriasis, which can damage the nails, often causes them to thicken, darken, and pit. Nail psoriasis is the medical term for this issue.

8. Pain, swelling, and stiffness in the joints are all symptoms of psoriatic arthritis, a condition that develops in some people with psoriasis.

9. Guttate psoriasis is characterized by the appearance of tiny, drop-shaped lesions on the skin, most frequently following a streptococcal infection. Compared to plaque psoriasis, these lesions are less severe and thinner.

10. Plaques with inverse psoriasis tend to show up in creases of skin, like the armpits, groin, and chest. Even if these don't produce scales, the constant rubbing of skin against skin can make them exceedingly painful and inflamed.

11. Erythrodermic psoriasis is a severe form of psoriasis characterized by widespread skin redness, skin peeling, and acute itching. Dehydration and infection are just two of the potential side effects.

The severity and duration of symptoms might vary greatly from one individual to the next. The physical manifestations of psoriasis are important, but the emotional and social effects can be just as devastating to a person's well-being. You should see a doctor or dermatologist if you have any reason to suspect you have psoriasis or are experiencing any of the condition's symptoms. Because of the chronic nature of psoriasis, treatment focuses on symptom management and control.

Psoriasis is diagnosed using a combination of a healthcare provider's examination of the affected area(s), a review of the patient's medical history, and, in some situations, further diagnostic procedures. Differential diagnosis, the process of eliminating potential alternative skin disorders, may also be performed. **Here is a rundown of the diagnostic process for psoriasis and the other skin**

disorders that may be considered:

• **Clinical Exam:** A dermatologist or other medical professional will examine the affected skin, looking for red plaques covered in silvery scales, the telltale sign of psoriasis. They will think about how these plaques will be placed and displayed.

• The patient's medical background is very important. Psorias is a skin ailment that can be helped by knowing about any relevant family history, previous skin conditions, drugs, infections, or traumas.

• A skin biopsy is a procedure that may be used in certain scenarios. A little piece of the damaged skin is removed for further analysis under the microscope. A biopsy can help rule out other skin disorders and confirm the diagnosis.

• A dermatologist may also look for signs of the Koebner phenomenon, in which psoriasis appears in places where the skin has been injured.

Psoriasis is one of several skin illnesses that can look similar, therefore it's crucial to rule out the alternatives throughout the diagnosis process.

1. Eczema (also known as atopic dermatitis) is a skin condition characterized by inflammation and itchiness but without the silvery scales typical of psoriasis. The severity and spread of the rash are two distinguishing factors.

2. Seborrheic dermatitis typically manifests itself on the scalp, face, and upper chest because these areas contain a high concentration of sebaceous glands. It can look similar to psoriasis but often lacks the dense scales observed in psoriasis.

3. Pityriasis rosea is a skin rash that appears as pink, scaly oval spots.

One enormous "herald patch" may appear first, followed by several smaller ones. Guttate psoriasis is a possible misdiagnosis.

4. Fungal infections, including ringworm (tinea), can cause rashes that seem like psoriasis but are actually round, red, and scaly. Differentiating psoriasis from fungal diseases requires a KOH test or culture.

5. Itchy, flat-topped, purple or brown papules or lumps are typical of the skin condition known as lichen planus. Due to its similarity in appearance to psoriasis, it is often misdiagnosed.

6. When an irritant or allergen comes into touch with the skin, it can cause a rash known as contact dermatitis. It can appear similar to psoriasis but is caused by a different process.

7. Mycosis fungoides is a very uncommon cutaneous T-cell lymphoma that, in its early stages, might look like psoriasis. Sometimes a biopsy is the only way to tell the difference.

To ensure a proper diagnosis and subsequent treatment, differential diagnosis is essential. Psoriasis can be distinguished from other skin conditions based on the dermatologist's assessment, the patient's clinical presentation, and, if necessary, the results of a biopsy. See a doctor or dermatologist if you think you have psoriasis or skin problems to get a proper diagnosis and tailored treatment plan.

CHAPTER THREE
Alternative Therapies for Psoriasis

Although psoriasis is incurable, there are several effective treatments that can be used to control the disease and its symptoms. The choice of treatment relies on the kind, intensity, and location of psoriasis, as well as individual characteristics. There are several main types of psoriasis treatments available today.

1. Localized Therapies:

• In mild to moderate psoriasis, anti-inflammatory creams or ointments containing corticosteroids are often used to alleviate symptoms like itching, redness, and inflammation.

Creams and ointments containing retinoid, a form of vitamin A, have been shown to inhibit cell proliferation and inflammation in the skin.

• Psoriasis on sensitive parts like the face and genitalia can be treated with immunosuppressive lotions or ointments called calcineurin inhibitors.

Preparations made from coal tar have been shown to alleviate psoriasis symptoms by lowering inflammation and delaying the proliferation of skin cells.

• **Topical Vitamin D Analogues:** These substances assist regulate skin cell proliferation and can be used to treat psoriasis.

2. The Use of Light in Treatment:

• **UVB Phototherapy**: Ultraviolet B (UVB) light exposure has been shown to inhibit cellular proliferation and reduce inflammation. It is frequently combined with topical therapies.

Combining a light-sensitizing drug (psoralen) with exposure to UVA light is the basis of a treatment known as PUVA (Psoralen plus UVA). For severe psoriasis, this is the treatment of choice.

3. Drugs Given Intravenously:

• In severe cases of psoriasis, your doctor may recommend oral retinoids to limit the proliferation of skin cells.

Psoriasis can be managed with the immunosuppressant methotrexate by decreasing inflammation and delaying the skin's cellular turnover rate.

• **Cyclosporine:** Another immunosuppressant, cyclosporine is administered for a limited time only for severe instances of psoriasis due to the risk of side effects.

Newer drugs, such as TNF-alpha inhibitors, IL-17 inhibitors, and IL-23 inhibitors, are available to treat psoriasis, and they work by blocking specific parts of the immune system. They are often reserved for more serious conditions.

4. Care for the Whole Body:

• Acitretin, a vitamin A-related oral drug, can suppress skin cell proliferation in psoriasis.

5. Therapies That Work Together:

To properly manage psoriasis, it may be necessary to employ a mix of treatments.

6. Healthful Habits and Self-Care:

• Moisturizing: Keeping the skin well-hydrated with moisturizers can help decrease irritation and scaling.

• Take a warm (not hot) bath with Epsom salts or colloidal oatmeal to calm your skin.

The symptoms can be controlled by avoiding the causes of them, such as stress, smoking, or certain drugs.

7. Consumption of Nutrients:

• Although there is no known cure for psoriasis, some people have found that making changes to their diet, such as cutting back on sugar and alcohol, has helped alleviate their symptoms.

8. Complementary and alternative medicine:

• Natural cures like aloe vera, fish oil, or capsaicin (found in chili peppers) may be appealing to some people, but it's important to talk to your doctor before trying anything new.

The choice of treatment should be chosen in consultation with a dermatologist or healthcare professional, taking into account the kind and severity of psoriasis, the individual's medical history, and any potential adverse effects. In order to get the best outcomes from treating psoriasis, treatment programs may need to be modified over time.

Nutritional Diet

Diet and nutrition can play a part in controlling psoriasis, although it's important to realize that there is no one-size-fits-all diet that works for everyone with the condition. The association between nutrition and psoriasis can vary from person to person because the condition is complex and multifactorial. But here are some nutritional things to think about that may help people with psoriasis:

• Foods Low in Inflammation Eating a diet high in anti-inflammatory foods has been linked to a decrease in psoriasis-related inflammation.

Fatty fish (salmon, mackerel), turmeric, ginger, nuts, and seeds (flaxseed, chia seeds), and so on should all find their way into your daily diet.

• Fish and certain plant foods, such as flaxseeds and walnuts, are good sources of omega-3 fatty acids, which are anti-inflammatory and may alleviate psoriasis symptoms.

• Vitamins, minerals, and antioxidants found in a diet rich in fruits and vegetables help maintain healthy skin and an effective immune system. Among these are blueberries, strawberries, spinach, kale, and sweet potatoes.

• Chicken, turkey, fish, beans, lentils, and tofu are all great lean protein options that you should include in your diet. Protein is essential for proper cell function and tissue repair.

• **Fiber-Rich Foods:** Foods high in fiber, such as whole grains, legumes, and vegetables, might help maintain a healthy gut flora, which may have a good impact on psoriasis.

• A healthy gut and immune system can be supported by eating probiotic-rich foods like yogurt or taking a probiotic supplement.

- **Drink Plenty of Water:** Adequate hydration is crucial for general health and can aid in maintaining supple skin.

- Restrict your alcohol intake, as doing so might exacerbate psoriasis symptoms and decrease the efficacy of some treatments. Please drink responsibly if you decide to imbibe.

- Some patients with psoriasis discover that eating particular foods, such processed foods, sugary snacks, or gluten-containing goods, might bring on or worsen their symptoms. Be aware of how various foods affect your body and think about cutting them out if necessary.

10. Get plenty of various nutrients from a wide variety of food groups and aim for a balanced and diverse diet. This may be beneficial to your physical and mental wellbeing.

It's vital to note that dietary modifications may take time to show an effect, and results can vary from person to person. If you have unique dietary needs, allergies, or health issues, talking to your doctor or a qualified dietitian before making any major changes to your diet is recommended.

Psoriasis therapy plans that include dietary changes should also include other treatments and modifications to the patient's lifestyle. Working with medical experts to develop a thorough strategy for treating your psoriasis should be your top priority.

CHAPTER FOUR
Managing Life with Psoriasis

Living with psoriasis can be hard, as it's a chronic condition that can impair not only your skin but also your whole well-being. It is possible to live a happy and successful life, though, with the right kind of management and some tweaks to one's routine. Here are some suggestions and things to think about if you have psoriasis:

• Get checked out by a dermatologist or other medical professional who has experience treating psoriasis. Effective management requires regular checkups and open communication with your healthcare team.

- **Adherence to Treatment:** Consistently use your prescribed treatment. Medications, UV therapy, biologic medicines, and topical therapies are all possibilities. Treatment regimen adherence is critical for symptom management.

- **Methods of Daily Living:**

Reducing Stress: Anxiety and worry can make psoriasis symptoms worse. To better handle stress, try some relaxation practices like yoga, deep breathing, or mindfulness meditation.

Even while there isn't a diet designed specifically for people with psoriasis, eating a nutritious, well-balanced diet can help improve health in general. Reducing one's intake of sugary drinks and alcoholic beverages may help alleviate symptoms for some people.

Exercising regularly is recommended for many health benefits, including stress relief, elevated mood, and longer life expectancy. Select physical activities that don't irritate your skin or joints.

Determine what makes your psoriasis flare up and steer clear of those situations in the future. Things including diet, medication, smoking, and the natural surroundings may all play a role.

• **Maintenance of the Skin:**

Moisturize frequently to prevent dryness and irritation caused by dehydration.

Take warm (not hot) baths or showers with light soap. Putting in skin-calming ingredients like Epsom salts or colloidal oatmeal.

• Select soft, breathable, and non-irritating fabrics for clothing to reduce the risk of chafing and discomfort. Clothing that fits loosely can also help, especially in regions affected by inverse psoriasis.

• Connect with individuals who understand what it's like to live with psoriasis by joining a support group. The support of others who can relate to your situation and learn from your story is invaluable.

• Educate yourself as much as can on psoriasis. Being able to make educated decisions about your care depends on knowing as much as possible about your condition, its causes, and the options for treating it.

- Maintaining a Healthy Body Image and Positive Self-Perception: Psoriasis. Keep in mind that your skin condition is not who you are. Focus on your abilities, passions, and the things that make you distinct.

- Visit your doctor often because psoriasis has been linked to other diseases like psoriatic arthritis and heart problems. Visiting your doctor regularly allows them to keep an eye on your health and treat any issues as they arise.

- Awareness and Advocacy Help psoriasis advocacy groups spread the word and end the discrimination people with the condition face. Psoriasis sufferers whose voices are heard through advocacy efforts see an increase in services and funding.

Maintaining a high quality of life while dealing with psoriasis can be challenging, but it is attainable with the right approach to treatment. Consider reaching out to healthcare providers and local support groups for assistance if you're dealing with psoriasis.

Conclusion

Psoriasis is a long-term skin disorder wherein red, scaly plaques form due to the fast proliferation of skin cells. Psoriasis's specific cause is unknown, however it is thought to entail a combination of genetics, environment, and immune system dysfunction.

- Several types of psoriasis exist, each with its unique set of symptoms and appearance on the skin: plaque psoriasis, guttate psoriasis, inverse psoriasis, pustular psoriasis, and erythrodermic psoriasis. For effective identification and care, a correct diagnosis and differential diagnosis are required.

• The degree and kind of psoriasis affect how it is treated. Treatment options range from external applications to whole-body drugs and behavioral adjustments. Although psoriasis can make day-to-day life difficult, it is possible to live a full and productive life with the correct approach to self-care and social support.

Working together with medical professionals, such as dermatologists, to create a treatment plan tailored to your needs and symptoms is essential.

Psoriasis sufferers can enhance their quality of life by learning as much as they can about the condition, finding healthy ways to deal with stress, and sticking to a routine of regular exercise.

Psoriasis is a chronic skin illness without a cure; nevertheless, new treatments and improved methods of care give people with the disease hope for improved quality of life.

THE END